# AUTISM IS AWESOME

RACHEL ELL

In this book, I will take you through everything from the ups and downs of being autistic. Firstly, there is nothing wrong with being autistic. I myself, 18 at the time of this book, was diagnosed last year and I am so grateful for my diagnosis.

What you can expect from this book.

This book covers everything from everyday struggles to signs and symptoms of autism to break it down for both adults, parents and children.

Disclaimer

Please do not use this book as a diagnostic tool. This book is purely to spread awareness and as a guide to children and families who have a diagnosis of autism.

# Contents

## What is Autism?

Autism is a Neurological Condition which affects communication and social skills. A neurological condition just means that your brain works differently than some others. That means you are Unique :).

Your social skills include being able to be an active listener for example making eye contact, which many people with autism struggle with. You may also find if you are autistic that you struggle to cooperate with other people meaning in group work activities you may be reluctant to hear other ideas for the project.

You are born with autism and there is no cure, but it can be managed with tools and strategies as you get older.

Autism can develop from genetics which means you may be born with autism if someone in your family has it. But parents, please don't blame yourself. It can also be caused by non-genetic factors. At least 1 in every 100 people in Scotland are autistic so it is more common than you think.

Autism may not be spotted at birth and the first years of life but later during the toddler or adolescent stage.
Remember symptoms are different for everyone so it can sometimes be hard to spot.

Sometimes the school or nursery that your child goes to will pick up on autism and advise you to see a doctor. If you are a parent, there is nothing to be ashamed of if you didn't see it yourself. In fact, I applaud you for seeing your child as they are.

Autism varies from person-to-person eg high-functioning or low-functioning autism. A person with low-functioning autism may be non-verbal or need one-on-one support with an adult where children with high-functioning autism are more able to do things for themselves.

Although your child may be high functioning, please don't feel like you can't get support for them. Everyone should get support high functioning or not.

Having autism can mean that you see and experience the world differently. It can mean that senses are heightened making going to a public place can be overwhelming or even having sensory-safe clothes to wear because the fabric doesn't irritate them.

For me, I get overwhelmed after a day out due to all the sensory input. If your child is like this consider letting them relax for the rest of the night and provide them with tools such as a fidget toy or a weighted blanket to calm them. A day like this may cause a meltdown. This is where your child may become violent and aggressive or cry because of everything from the day being built up.

## Signs

So, what exactly are the signs of Autism? Autism has a broad range of signs and symptoms to look out for, but some are easier to spot. Let me break it down for you into two sections. Preschool (0-5yr) and school age (5+)

Preschool

One sign of autism in the preschool range is your child not responding to their name. A neurotypical baby should be able to respond quite easily to their name by the time they turn one. If you notice your child not responding it could be autism. A child with autism may not value social interactions even at that age, which can cause them to not respond.

A baby with autism may not be interested or react to faces. Autistic children have a hard time recognising facial features or expressions so they may not understand why you are smiling at them.

Avoiding eye contact can be spotted at this age however is usually present throughout childhood. In a conversation you may catch your child avoiding eye contact. This could be because they are avoiding negative affective arousal which is emotions such as sadness, disgust and anger.

In a recent study, some adults with autism said they experience adverse emotional responses and feel invaded with eye contact. This also explains wanting to avoid negative affective arousal.

An autistic child can get very upset if they don't like the texture or smell of something. Autism can cause heightened senses which means some unfamiliar textures or smells can cause an overstimulation and be too much for them. Remember your child is experiencing senses that are stronger than most! It's their superpower.

## School Age

Older children with autism may but into conversations or talk over other people. Autistic people can find it hard to understand the concept of waiting their turn to speak or have a go at something. Remember, your child is not rude they just can't understand it properly :)

Your child may have a special interest and you may find them talking about it a lot. This is because children may find greater rewards/pleasure out of non-social stimuli than a social stimuli as it is much easier for a child to understand.

Most autistic children have an adverse reaction to change. They may become aggressive or withdrawn when being told that their routine is going to change. Children prefer similar environments that are sensory-safe and have no surprises.

A new place or situation can be extremely stressful for an autistic person with their heightened senses and the anxiety of meeting new people. For example, a child may be experiencing anxiety from having to change schools. They have new people to meet who don't know them. They are in an unfamiliar environment with no routine and no sense of security.

Finally, some children with autism find it very hard to understand what or how others are feeling. For example, if a child is upset about a toy, a person with autism may not understand that that toy that has been lost is very important to them.

In a more subtle way, autistic children can find it hard to recognise a change in body language or tone of voice. If a child is sad, we usually pick up that their voice is softer or a bit shaky however someone with autism may not pick up on that change and not comfort the child who is sad.

# Mimicking

Have you caught your child or yourself even, copying other people's body language and tone or even speak in a different accent after watching TV?

I have and this is called mimicking. Mimicking in autism is when you imitate something you have seen or heard and people my mimic because in that situation that is the norm. The way you are meant to act. The rules.

Mimicking in autism can be seen as imitating (copying) physical actions, such as clapping, facial expressions and reactions.

Think of a chain reaction. Someone is upset and crying and their emotions cause someone else to cry, then you start crying. That is mimicking. So actually, it is more common than you think.

This is more common in adolescents as children with autism may find it harder to pick up emotions/reactions and be interested in others. It is a lot easier for adolescents to mimic as they have a better understanding of the world and observe other people more closely.

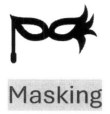

Masking

In this world full of different people with different personalities you might be surprised to find that there are more people with autism than you think. This may be due to masking. Did you know, around 700,000 uk citizens have autism?

So, if no one has explained masking to you, I will. Masking is where a neurodiverse child will cover up and change the way they act around certain people to hide their condition.
   Some people may feel like they have to hide it in order to fit in or be included.
It may also include mimicking others to appear neurotypical.

Masking is different for everyone but some examples of masking in children and teens with autism are making eye contact and mimicking a neurotypical's body language.

Children can mask in other ways as well, here are some detailed examples of how a child masks.

A child may suppress soothing behaviours such as stimming which are repetitive movements that calm a child. Although normal to the autistic child, others may think it's weird so in order to be seen as "normal" a child me feel the need to stop doing them to avoid judgement from others.

Another example is that a neurodiverse child may create scripts or go over conversations in their head to use in social situations. These are like a checklist for the child to use in social situations to appear neurotypical.

A child who masks may be very tired, angry or upset after masking in public. This is because masking uses a lot of energy. Think of it like acting. A child who has autism needs to play the role of a neurotypical child. They are bound to get tired!

This can cause a meltdown due to pent-up emotions from the day. Autistic people can find it hard to understand their emotions, so this is to be expected after masking. A child may also have a meltdown because they are tired and frustrated.

## Stimming

Stimming is a self-soothing behaviour, usually repetitive, used by neurodiverse people. Stimming can help ground a person in stressful situations or help them express feelings of happiness or excitement. This is because stimming can distract an autistic person from feeling these big emotions or take away from a situation they are uncomfortable in.

It is usually a repetitive movement or noises, and autistic children can start stimming at any age. It can vary in intensity for children and teens. Some might need to stim more frequently than others with autism and can have bigger stims like rocking or hand flapping whereas other children may just tap or flick their fingers.

## Signs of Stimming

Spinning – Spinning in a child with autism is usually a stim. Your child may run in circles until they get dizzy or twirl when they play their favourite song. It could mean that your child may need more sensory input and a space to stim in a safe area that ensures they won't get hurt, or hurt anyone else, when spinning.
Rocking – You may notice your child rock back and forth when sitting down. This may be due to your child being upset or needing stimulation.

This type of stimming is usually harmless and can help your child relax.
Visual stimming – Visual stimming is when a child uses their eyes to get a sensory input. They may blink hard or repetitively (one of my stims) or gaze at moving or glistening objects such as a fan spinning or, looking at jewellery and ornaments that sparkle. This sort of visual satisfaction relaxes an autistic child.

Although swimming is usually harmless, there are some self-injurious stims to look out for like punching or biting themselves.

One thing to note is that there are ways around self-injurious stimming. For example, if your child is stimming because they need more stimulation, then you can provide materials such as a sensory swing or weighted blankets/ vest *etc*. This will satisfy most sensory seekers needs.

Another way of helping a sensory seeker is to do massages and pressure point stimulation before school or event. This can relax your child, so they are less likely to experience a meltdown. Massages can help regulate their sensory system. This also creates a bond between you and your child.

## Sensory Sensations

Due to the differences in an autistic child's brain, there is no surprise that they might see the world in a different way than neurotypical peers. One of thing that plays a big role in experiencing the world is our 5 senses.

Taste, touch, smell, sight and hearing can all be affected by autism.

Firstly, have you ever noticed that your child with autism has aversions, this is because autism increases all your senses to the max. Children might not like certain foods that have strong flavours like sausage or pepperoni because the flavour is far too strong in their minds.

This is also the case. for textures. Foods might be too crunchy, slimy or rough for them to enjoy.

Generally speaking, when an autistic child doesn't like a certain texture or taste, they are repulsed by it.

On a similar note, smells can overpower an autistic child, sometimes even more than taste! Imagine you are cooking, the house fills with the "pleasant" smell of spag ball, however your child is complaining that the smell is awful and is completely consuming them and all they can think about is that smell.

One interesting thing that is more common in autistic people is that strong smells can give them a headache. I can vouch for this as I too get headaches as a result of a strong fragrance.

Bright lights can be troublesome for an autistic person. Due to hypersensitivity, bright lights can cause eye pain and headaches. With added glare or LED'S in an already stimulating environment, it can be hard to process visual stimuli.

Finally, an autistic child hearing is superior but it's not always a good thing. A child with autism may be able to hear a hum coming from the fridge or static from the computer. It can distract them and cause them to lose focus.

They may get angry or have a meltdown because they are annoyed due to the repetitive sound or frustrated because they don't understand where the sound is exactly coming from or how to stop it.

## Schools and Nurseries

There is no doubt in saying that being neurodivergent in school and nursery can be stressful, aggravating and downright hard.

Firstly, there's socialising. Children are expected to make friends and socialise from a very young age. Think of all the toddler groups, all the birthdays you took your child to. Socialising starts early and that can be hard for someone who is autistic.

Nurseries can be challenging for people at the best of times, but autism can make it harder. One thing being lack of routine. Although nurseries are trying to implement schedules, there is no one set activity. Nursery's expect children to choose their activity and too much choice can be a struggle for autistic youngsters.

Something I found hard in school was suppressing my stimming. I'm not going to lie it is sometimes embarrassing. On my way to class, where it was busy, I would get all my energy out. If I needed to stim in class, I found it helpful to do less noticeable things like looking at lights or tapping my fingers together.

Finally, exams. Exams can be hard for an autistic person. They are usually in a big hall with hundreds of other students all working at the same time, there's coughing, kicking, you name it.

It can be very distracting and agitating. That's why most schools offer separate accommodation which can be a private room. This can be extremely helpful for older children.

For both nursery and school-aged children, making, and keeping friends can be difficult. Children with autism often lack social skills meaning their interactions with other children are difficult.

A child with autism may not make eye contact or seem uninterested in the conversation causing the other child to feel unimportant.

Also, something a lot of neurodivergents do is assume that everyone else knows what they are talking about. This can cause tension as it seems so impossible that their friend doesn't know about the topic they are really passionate in. This makes them feel emotions like frustration or anger that they can't understand.

## Autism Annoyances

Now although autism is nothing to be ashamed of nor a bad thing, there are some annoyances that come with autism so I thought I would share some!

No. 1 – You can't sit still during a film. Now I find when I'm sitting watching a film, I cannot sit still for the life of me. It is like torture. I can feel every bone in my body, every hair, my skin you name it and I just feel the need to stim to stop me from wriggling like a child. It is purely like an itch you can't scratch. And the worst thing is that you moving and stimming annoys other people, so it is a lose lose situation.

No. 2 – We sometimes (possibly a lot of the time) don't get jokes/sarcasm. This is a known one but it's true. Sometimes a non-autistic person will make a joke and it just doesn't click in an autistic person's brain. I find this especially the case when the joke is about me. I just don't get it.

No.3 – Hating tags, now this is a common one. I personally hate tags on clothes, they are itchy and annoying, but I also hate them when they are cut off. It's worse than being left on as you are constantly being scratched by a rough piece of fabric every time you move. Why can we not win?

No. 4 – We randomly understand something hours or days after. I could literally be in bed and understand a joke that was said earlier in the day. It will just get me at the most random times.

No. 5 – We annoy people which annoys us. I get it we can sometimes be annoying with our stims or speaking for hours about our special interest but to us it is important, and we don't understand that we annoy others.

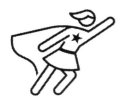

## Superpowers With Autism

To end this book, let's go over some superpowers that comes with having autism.

There is a lot of gifts/talents that come with autism, and it is always nice to reflect on them to remind yourself how awesome you are!

Firstly, creativity. People with autism are extremely creative. They are often into crafts, writing or reading. It is really positive to see the talent in lots of young children with autism. It is important to develop their skills by providing creative outlets each day.

People on the spectrum have exceptional memory. We can remember things in extreme detail years after it happened. In fact, a lot of children with autism could give you an exact run down of their birthday last year.

High intellectual ability is possible in older autistic children. It can be due to faster brain growth a good memory. Some autistic children and teens have a high focus helping improve their knowledge.

## Tips From an Autistic

First tip, never give up on supporting your child. They need you; they rely on you to help them with day-to-day life. Don't give up because you are frustrated and tired of the meltdowns and reactions. Stay strong for them.

Second, plan time each day to bond with your child. For example, if they are into trains have time to play with the trains together. Bonding with your child over their interests shows them that you care and also promotes language skills as you talk about the activity.

if your child is nonverbal, make sure to speak to them a lot. Read them stories and reinforce what they are asking for. Overtime your child may start saying a few words and make progress in development.

Use your child's name so they know and learn to respond to it. This is hugely beneficial for school and nursery as their name will be used by many staff and peers, so it is important to build up the skill of responding to their name as soon as possible.

## About the Author

Rachel Ell is an ambitious young adult writer from Scotland. She is always looking to be doing something creative.

Rachel was diagnosed with autism in January 2023 and chose to write this book as an honour to all the autistic children out there with the hopes of getting autism some acceptance.

I aim to make my writing inclusive and friendly for anyone to read. I personally don't like it when books are wordy and hard to understand and, in my books, you won't get that.

Reminder – You are enough. It does not matter, autistic or not, everyone deserves to be.

Printed in Great Britain
by Amazon

28680367R10015